Rapid Weight Loss Hypnosis

Self-Hypnosis for Burning Fat, Losing Weight Naturally, and Living Healthy, Including Positive Affirmations and Meditations

DIANA WILLIAMS

RapidWeightLossHypnosis

DISCLAIMER

Weight loss results vary from person to person. This book is not intended as a substitute for the medical advice of physicians. The reader should regularly consult a physician in matters relating to his/her health and particularly with respect to any symptoms that may require diagnosis or medical attention. The content on this book is for informational purposes only.

Table of Contents

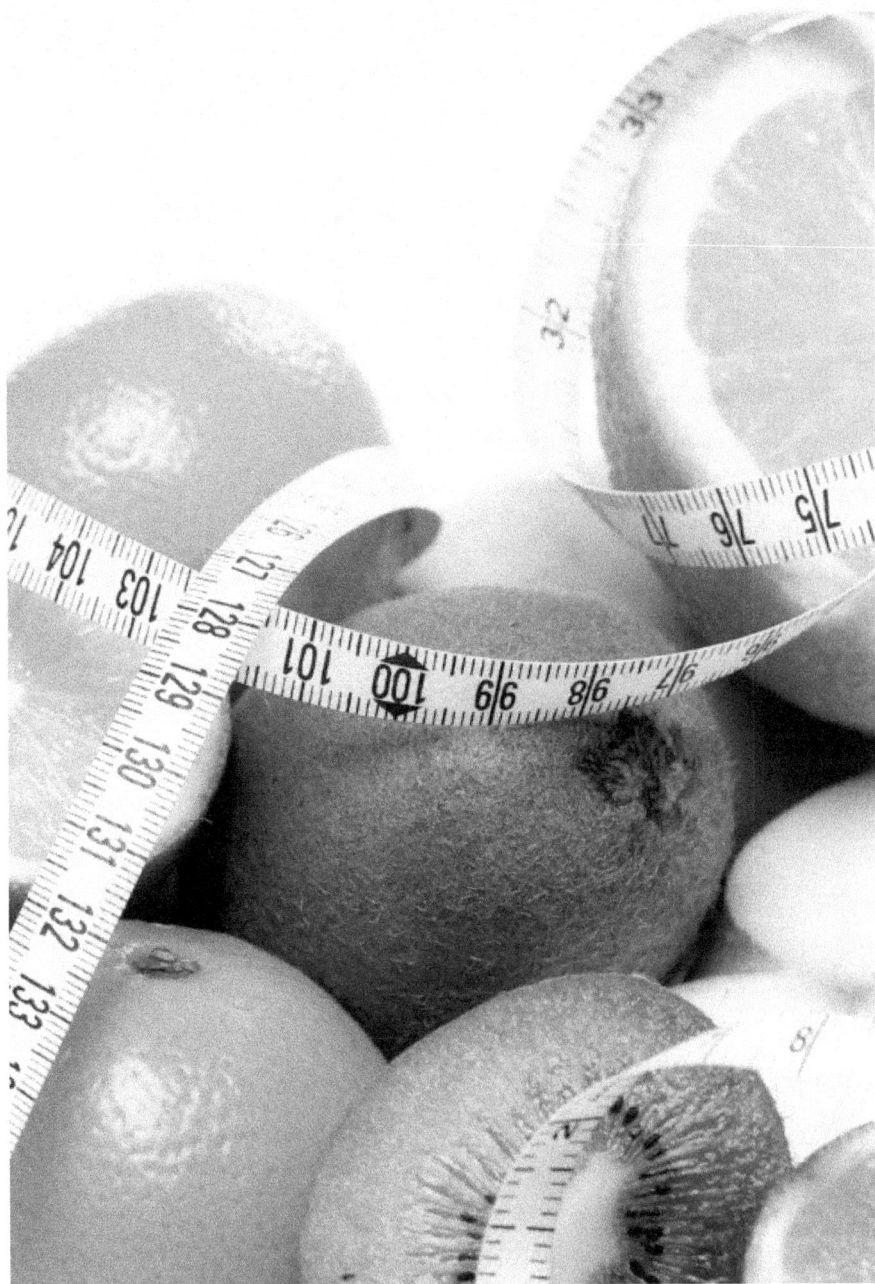

Introduction

Y ou look in the mirror, and you are dissatisfied. Do you wish that your shape, nose, legs, and hair were like somebody else's? Why do we always compare ourselves?

Why aren't we reconciled with our appearance? We heard disgusting, even though we have mistaken or defects, we should still love ourselves.

It includes things related to our personality as well as our bodies. It is not about not wanting to change. It is a commendable endeavor to achieve or retain their looks or care about looking more attractive.

At the same time, most people are much more critical, stricter with themselves than justified.

They are continuously dissatisfied with themselves and don't see in the mirror what others see.

Some girls feel very uncomfortable when looking at each other. They generally don't like looking at each other because they don't like what they see. Where did these reactions come from?

Usually, you don't look at yourself; you only see yourself concerning that ideal of beauty that you have in your head. It is where dissatisfaction creeps in. We compare ourselves with those we consider better than ourselves; self-esteem is negatively affected. We all have a model in the head, a term of comparison that we have built by looking at years of magazines, advertising, and movies with perfect Hollywood princesses.

The mantra must become one and only one: there is no need to compare me to that model because everybody is a unique, generous specimen, rich in the indications of what I am.

If we can accept our own life, life will become simpler and happier.

After all, if we focus our attention on what is terrible, we reinforce the bad. And what we pay the most attention to as we think about something will come true.

That's why you are unique. Be happy that you are different from anyone, that you look the way you do and that it is just you. Start to feel that it's your own body, not something separate you need to live with.

Do you love the little things that carry memories? Don't you love the atmosphere of your messy place after playing with your kids?

How should you love your body?

Sandra Díaz Ferrer, a researcher at the University of Granada, works with women who do not like their bodies and suffer from eating disorders. Imagine you have a fear of bugs that obsesses you. The psychologist might ask you to look closely at bugs until you get used to them, desensitizing yourself to the features that first terrified you. You can apply the same procedure to your body (Ferrer, 2015).

Here are some ways to cultivate enormous gratitude in everyday life. When faced with a negative situation, do not be discouraged. Ask yourself instead what you can learn for the future and for reasons to feel grateful.

Promise yourself not to be hostile or not to criticize yourself for three days. This exercise will help you understand that negative thoughts are just a waste of energy. Every day, list the reasons why you feel grateful. The body is a miracle, and you should celebrate all the gifts it has given you. Take note of it every day. Go to the next body part and do the same.

When you have reached your toes, return to your head again, to your face, and now, going downhill, just say to all your body parts, "I love you." Even if you feel a little stupid about it, don't stop. You see, you're going to have a completely different relationship with your appearance. And by the way, let's not forget, it's not a coincidence that it's called outer. What's inside is more important. But what's inside is visible outside.

Use your inner self to love your outer, and you will be much calmer, happier, more satisfied, and more confident.

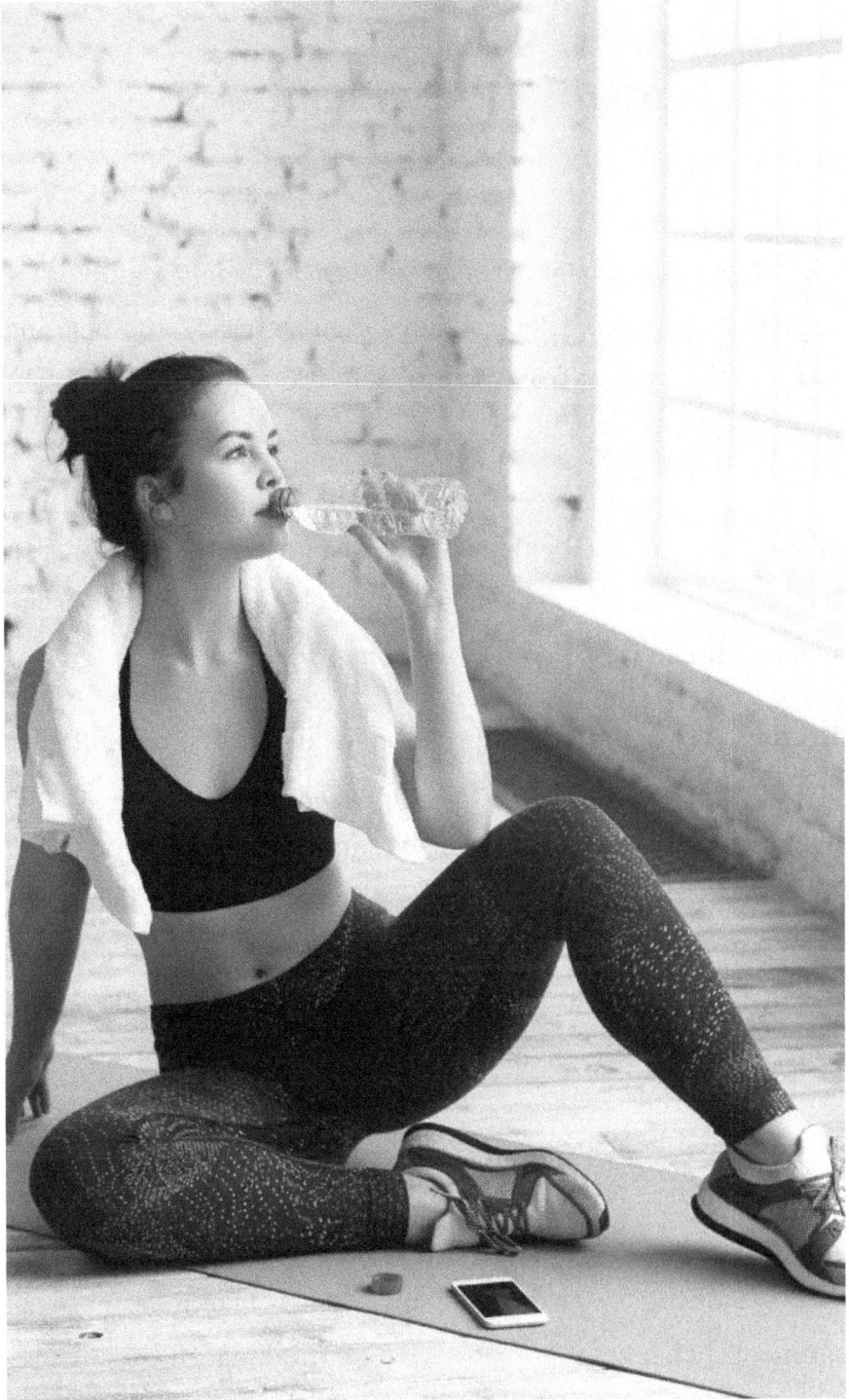

Chapter 1.
Mind-Body Practices

People who experience disease, accidents and other trauma to their bodies often react by dissociating themselves from painful sensations and physical self-awareness.

While this can be beneficial in the short term, it can also conflict with a person's ability to self-regulate and create meaningful behavioral improvements.

Obesity is a source of depression in itself, and weight loss consumers still detach from their bodies-this This is one explanation that they can over-eat and not be aware of actual satiation signals. When it comes to patterns and behaviors that may not benefit the development of well-being in general, parts of the body may respond negatively, given the individual's conscious intention to do otherwise.

Our mission is not only to teach customers about their mind-body connectivity, which happens to be bi-directional but to help them become more adept at using it as a healing tool. Because of this two-way function, we can take a "top-down" approach, change a person's way of thinking and feeling to affect changes in their physiology, or take a "bottom-up" tact physical functions to improve the thoughts and emotional state of a person.

Another approach I help clients work towards enhancing their awareness and responding to their bodies' signals and building self-acceptance is to use a massage on the abdomen. This strategy will also help overcome stomach issues that encourage unhealthy eating and drinking, or even traumatic conditions.

The abdomen is genuinely an energy source, a powerhouse in itself. The Japanese call this center of our body "hara," a place where "ki," or energy, is produced. During my martial arts training, I learned to embrace and focus on this part of my body, and once I did, I broke through some previous mental and physical limitations.

Releasing unhelpful discomfort in the abdomen can relax the entire body and mind, with several positive outcomes resulting:

1) Reduces chronic stress and anxiety, and alleviates pain

2) Increases metabolism and enhances intestinal fires

3) Builds self-acceptance

4) Strengthens the connection between mind and body and increases awareness of physical sensations

Meditation for mindful hypnosis of the heart

For individual communities, like ours, people are admonished to "suck for your belly at a young age! "(Do you unintentionally keep stress in yours right now?!) Regardless of height and weight, we are full of self-awareness in this part of the body and feel inside. As a result, we are often detached from our heart and may have pessimistic feelings about it.

Even if a person doesn't struggle to be overweight, they can "keep" the gut unconsciously in a strengthened, restricted role. Practicing this belly exercise will make the enteric nervous system-the digestive tract-transition towards a "remembered health" more relaxed.

Sit quiet, with your eyes closed. Take your thoughts to the middle area, to your heart. Let yourself aware of how you feel about that part of your body. Let the emotions, concepts, and opinions rise into your consciousness, like bubbles flowing from the sea. Do not be your feelings; just watch them unfold. You can experience hearing your voice or hearing specific thoughts in someone else's voice as well. Just watch them as they float up.

You should count your breath as you breathe in, count as you catch your breath, and count as you breathe out. Using the diaphragm, you want to live heavily, and your abdomen inflates more than your chest region. It is a simple way to help the conscious mind shift away from disturbing or disruptive thoughts and activate relaxation. You might want to apply some imagery to it, including seeing a number written in sand, and seeing a gentle wave wash it away, replacing it with the next number. And, you can want to consider the numbers in your head.

Note when you do so that the stomach muscles are relaxed and other body muscles relax as they do. Just when your stomach settles, does it become possible to dissipate the pain in your body fades away? A surge of warmth passes over you and helps your mind to become calm, peaceful.

Then raise your right hand to the top of your uterus, gently resting it just below your bra line. Pressing gently, in a clockwise direction, start rotating it to the left. It should rub your belly's outer circumference gently, reaching up to the tops of the arms, falling to the bottom of the navel, and then reversing the other hand. Your skin and flesh move by gentle pressure but will not feel uncomfortable.

Imagine that as you massage your "hara," you activate and balance the life-force within you. You link inside this personal, intense center. When you find that there are troubling thoughts or emotions, let them float both up and down. Consider that something that blocks, inhibits, or otherwise harms you is being dislodged and discharged.

Begin to breathe deeply and rhythmically, inhale excellent, soothing substances, and exhale all that isn't beneficial or curative.

Imagine your healthy, fully working digestive tract, returned to optimal fitness. Bring in a state of peace a state of well-being just though you experience revitalization and regeneration of the energies within your heart.

When you've done 10-12 massage rotations, relax and indulge in the sensations of relaxation and calm now, realizing that you'll experience the good benefits of having this unique period as you return to your usual activities.

Spend a few minutes a day in abdominal yoga, and you will realize after a short time that not only the abdomen and overall body will feel better, but the digestive system will also change!

Body Parts

We may also use a method called "Body Parts" to enhance the connection between mind and body. This approach can be a stand-alone strategy, or it can quickly improve specifictechniques you use to assist a customer.

Ultimately it acts as an excellent method to attract and expand a customer for future research. It helps to build hope that you will "open the door" between a person's aware and subconscious minds, encouraging them to connect openly to aspects of themselves that will be part of a "unit" of recovery.

Start with inducing some consumer concentration and relaxation. You can make them concentrate on breathing; they can place their attention on a hand or leg, leading them to close their eyes and finding they can still imagine that portion of their body, even with their eyes closed. The key goal is to focus their attention on their physical self. Using something similar from here, like:

When you learn your side, now you may think about all the stuff the side does with you how it supports you in so many ways touching, stroking, squeezing, grabbing, raising, folding, feeding (describing every client-relevant tasks)

Abeautiful hand is a hand. I wonder if you should say it what you think of what it does for you?

PAUSE

So, if the hand were able to talk, what would it tell you? And what is it you need?

PAUSE

That's right and talk of your heart now, please the incredible pump the allows blood to circulate to keep you healthy.Yourwonderful heart, built to beat so many times in your lifetime. Nobody knows exactly how many cycles it is, but it works to achieve the beats for you. Who do you want your heart to tell?

PAUSE

So, what does the heart want to tell you about what it's going through about what you need? Hear it now.

PAUSE

That's right, and now just talk of your big toe on your left foot (* or some other, untouched part of your body, maybe an eyebrow or an ear). That's helping you keep calm to make you walk. Your beautiful big toe builds to help you make more strides in your life.

No one knows precisely how many steps this is, but it works to do the number of moves for you. I'm curious if you will let yourself be overwhelmed with admiration of how good the toe works for you and will continue to.

PAUSE

So, would the toe like to talk to (any part of the body which needs healing) now? Should this happen, what will they tell each other?

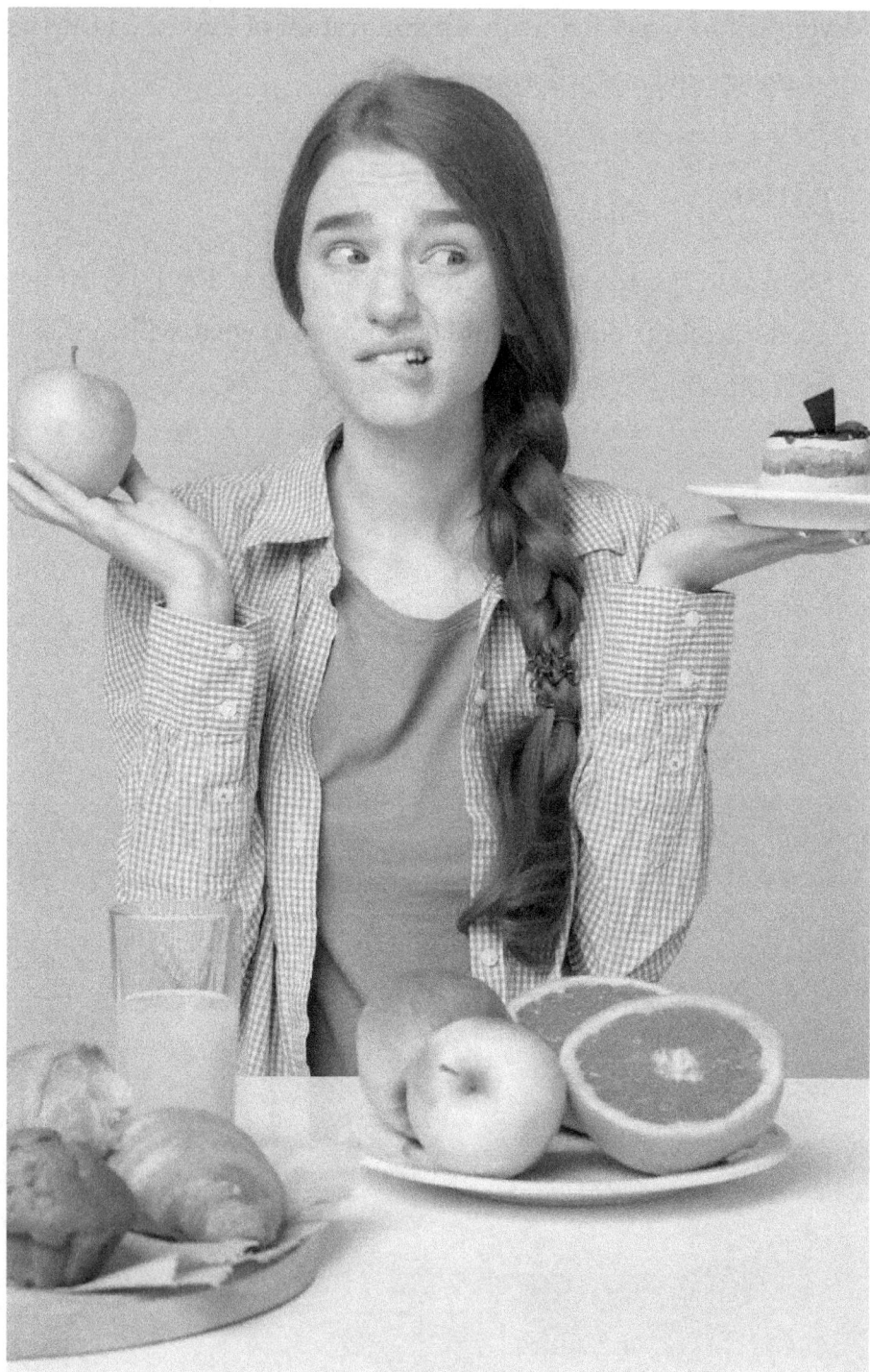

Chapter 2.
Stopping Food Addiction

Food is what we all depend on for survival, nourish us, cheer for us, and contribute to our health. In an ideal world, we would eat various balanced diets to satisfy us physically and emotionally.

However, sadly, food is a complicated topic.Some of us can establish unhealthy relationships with food, use it in unhelpful ways, and create a behavioral addiction in some cases.

Highly palatable foods (i.e., those high in fat, sugar, or salt) cause a chemical reaction within the brain, causing a sense of gratification and satisfaction.

This reaction can get addictive for anyone with an unhealthy food relationship. Although eating disorders are not known as "food addiction," this relationship with food can cause physical and psychological difficulties.

Here we will go deeper into the concept of food addiction and how hypnotherapy can help you develop a safer, happier relationship with food.

What is Addiction to Food?

There is a lot of controversy as to whether food addiction does exist in the catering industry. Brain imaging and other studies of people with 'food addictions' have shown similar outcomes to alcohol addictions.

Unlike drug addiction, however, food addiction is not a chemical dependency; it's a behavioral dependency.

Therefore, people are not addicted to food per se, but rather to the act of eating and the feeling they get after feeding. It appears to be improved by highly palatable foods, as they release feel-good chemicals, such as dopamine, into the brain.

People who develop this behavioral problem can be obsessed with food and eating thoughts. They can experience shameful feelings after eating too. Eating those foods also comes with a side of guilt due to our diet culture driven society and unrealistic beauty standards, making it very difficult for people to cultivate balanced and rational attitudes towards food.

What causes addiction to food?

Like in other addictions, there is never a single cause but rather a combination of reasons. It may be biological, psychological, or social influences. Physical causes include hormonal imbalances, a variation in the brain's development, side effects of other drugs, or even a family member dealing with addictions.

Psychological factors may include witnessing trauma or violence, difficulty coping with negative emotions, low self-esteem, or dealing with grief or loss when suffering mentally; food as a soothing mechanism or managing method.

If this is at the heart of your addiction, if you want to change your relationship with food, it's essential to fix it.

Certain aspects of mental wellbeing can also affect poor eating behaviors. These problems include eating disorders, anxiety, and depression.

Sometimes treatment can help you improve your relationship with food.

Social factors contributing to food addiction include family issues, peer or societal pressure, and feeling isolated and stressful events in life. Try to discuss and talk about your ideas in a support group or with friends and family.

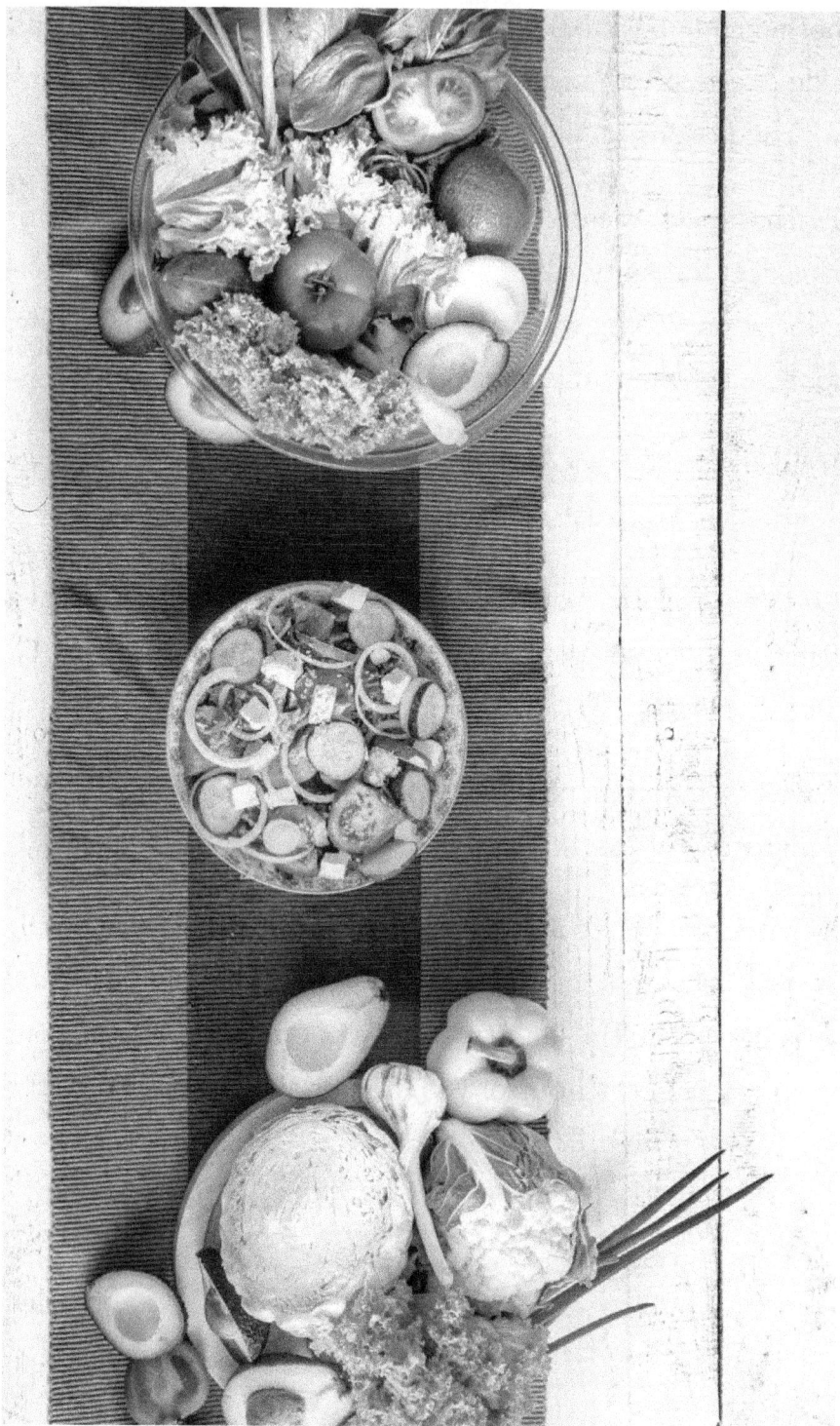

Chapter 3.
Portion Control

Here are some straightforward improvements you can consider yourself slim:

1. Toss out Your Scales

Do you think flimsy individuals bounce on the scales each morning? No, they don't. Fixating on the leaves makes you a captive to them. At the point when you lose a pound or two, you may feel extraordinary, yet if you increase a little, at that point, it can set you into a winding of implosion.

The sentiments of disappointment that pursue can send you running for the closest bar of chocolate or other solace nourishment.

Also, restroom scales are not a precise method to screen your weight. Imagine a scenario where you are practicing more and picking up muscle. Alternatively, perhaps you need a decent stable discharge—well, there goes a couple of additional pounds.

Women, it is that time, and your body puffs up with liquid weight. Such a large number of components can impact that number on the scales.

So, it's an excellent opportunity to quit deciding your prosperity by what you gauge and start taking a gander at all the positive changes you make in your life. Give you a chance to feel, and the sound decisions you make will be your new weight reduction indicator. Or on the other hand, essentially watch as your garments get looser and your body gets littler.

2. Tune in to Your Body

Pause for a minute or two to inquire as to whether you feel incredibly eager. There are when we think we feel hungry, however just a not many when we are willing.

Frequently we feed our sentiments as a result of a bogus enthusiastic craving. Or on the other hand, perhaps we ruin feeling anxious for feeling hungry.

Genuine hunger is a slight chewing or void sensation in your stomach. Set aside an effort to tune in to your body, to tune in to your body's needs truly. Eat possibly to fulfill genuine craving and stop when your body has had enough. Pick food sources that make you feel fulfilled, supported, and light and keep away from all nourishments that make you think substantial, enlarged, and awkward. It's as straightforward as that!

3. Bite Your Food

Processing starts in your mouth, and great assimilation is essential to changing the nourishment you eat into the vitality your body needs.

When you bite your food, it invigorates the discharge of stomach related catalysts in your stomach and stomach related tract.When you eat too rapidly, these proteins don't have the opportunity to process your nourishment viably.

When you eat quickly, you likewise swallow more air and ingest more significant parts of food, putting a strain on your stomach related framework and causing swelling and gas.

Additionally, the appetite hormone Leptin will keep on expanding as you eat until your hunger fulfills.

Biting your nourishment altogether and eating gives your body time to perceive that it is full and permits leptin to communicate something specific from your stomach to your cerebrum to quit eating since you have had enough.

4. Eat Smaller Meals More Often

Eat no less than every 4-5 hours to give your body the fuel it needs to work effectively. It will help keep up your glucose levels and keep your digestion firing up.

Always plan a nutritious diet as a goal, and remember that you only need to eat when you start to feel hungry, not when you are craving.When you experience over the top appetite, it indicates low glucose levels, which will make longings for sugar and other CRAP nourishments.

5. Make the most of Your Food

Plunk down, slow down, unwind and make the most of your nourishment. Making a loose and charming climate when you eat urges you to bite all the more completely, eat all the more gradually, and make it simpler to tune in to your body.

Likewise, attempt to abstain from whatever occupies your consideration away from nourishment, for example, sitting in front of the TV. Along these lines, you bind to stay mindful of the amount you are eating.

The more you understand when you eat, the more you will listen to slogans that indicate that you are full.

Tips to Stay Motivated

Indeed, even with the best program and all the help on the planet, we as a whole have days when we could utilize some additional motivation. To build your inspiration, here are a few things you can do and assurance your weight reduction achievement.

Set Achievable Goals

Something I can't pressure enough is the significance of making changes that you will have the option to stay with for a fantastic remainder.

First, define a short-term achievable goal, which is not attached to the numbers. For model, rather than making it your destination to lose 10 kilograms, why not intend to drink eight water glasses each day.

Or then again, plan to take the stairs every morning on your approach to work. Another very accommodating objective is to tune in to your charming chronicles, in any event, four times each week. Whatever your goals, ensure they are quite sure, unmistakable, and simple to achieve.

Move more actively is critical to well-being. When you try to lose weight, it brings unprecedented changes. Nevertheless, exhaustion with the conventional old exercise program is almost a difficult task for an extended period.Try not to stall out stuck!

Prepare for the New You

Prepare for the new form of yourself that you are making. Wipeout, any unfortunate nourishment from the cabinets, dispose of old garments from the wardrobe. Modify your condition to suit the new life you are building.

Try not to Give In to Guilt

The main thing amiss with the infrequent guilty pleasure is the blame you feel a short time later.

It doesn't help to make yourself feel so bad. One binge eating will make you entirely off track, and finally, eat ten chocolates to feel good.

Naturally, flimsy individuals don't feel regretful when they have a rare treat. They relish the experience and afterward get directly back to eating well nourishments. Blame isn't valuable—let it go!

Methodologies and Techniques for Reprogramming Yourself

Have you ever considered how to excel in certain things-exceed your job expectations and become an extraordinary partner and parent, but when it comes to knowing how to eat well, nothing is indeed organized and in shape? Regularly when we're not effective in specific regions, we're feeling the loss of some significant segment—some procedure or system that could support us.

We endeavor to tackle an issue with an answer that comes up short—and for reasons unknown, we can't come to an obvious conclusion and see that the arrangement isn't exactly working, or that we don't have an improved circumstance. Take what happens when we eat for enthusiastic reasons.

It's merely putting a bandage on an issue while simultaneously making new issues for us, including weight increase and sentiments of blame, disappointment, and being crazy.

A portion of these examples and methodologies will be shiny new to you, and others will be alterations of ones you're now utilizing.However, maybe you aren't using them very right. At that point, we'll investigate how to take these new examples and transform them into propensities-programmed programs that your mind executes without you pondering them any longer.

Healthy Food Hypnosis: Updating Your Habitual Programming

How to drive a vehicle? Do you recall how overpowering it was? Furthermore, what about how—do you consider moving similarly? After some time, we have a "program" inside our intuitive personality that realizes how to drive a vehicle. When we get into a car, that program can dominate and assist us with moving, so we don't need to consider it deliberately. We can call these projects propensities.

One of the most dominant ways mesmerizing causes us is by enlightening the propensities-programs we now have running. A portion of these projects does not help us—like the "I'm pushing, so I need to eat the dessert program."

Also, we need to supplant that program with a refreshed form,preferably—one that still fits the first wanted result's need without causing undesirable reactions (expanded weight addition and potential sentiments of blame and disappointment).

Up to this point, we've examined what I call the fundamental root issue—the psychological and passionate parts, including restricting convictions that keep us caught. You can think about that as the establishment of the work we do. Upon the establishment, there are parts of everyday life that are important to address also.

These angles are a tendency, whether fortunate or unfortunate, are based on the organization. Good spelling work is mostly a two-dimensional approach: we manage the hidden roots (organizations), and we do it every day.

Take a walk around work and life (everything depends on the establishment). We would prefer not just to take a gander at the routine segments since that gives a transitory fix. When we do both simultaneously, what happens is that we decidedly move how we feel inside, notwithstanding trading unfortunate propensities for sound maintainable ones. It works since what we are doing moves how we think, which gives the long-haul advantage and makes solid propensities that provide quick outcomes.

In neuroscience, which is the examination and capacity of the sensory system and cerebrum, there is a significant perspective that clarifies why propensities work called Hebb's Law. Hebb's Law expresses that whatever flames together, wires with regards to our mind and neurons. It implies that when we complete two things together (whatever loves together), they connect in our minds (wires together).

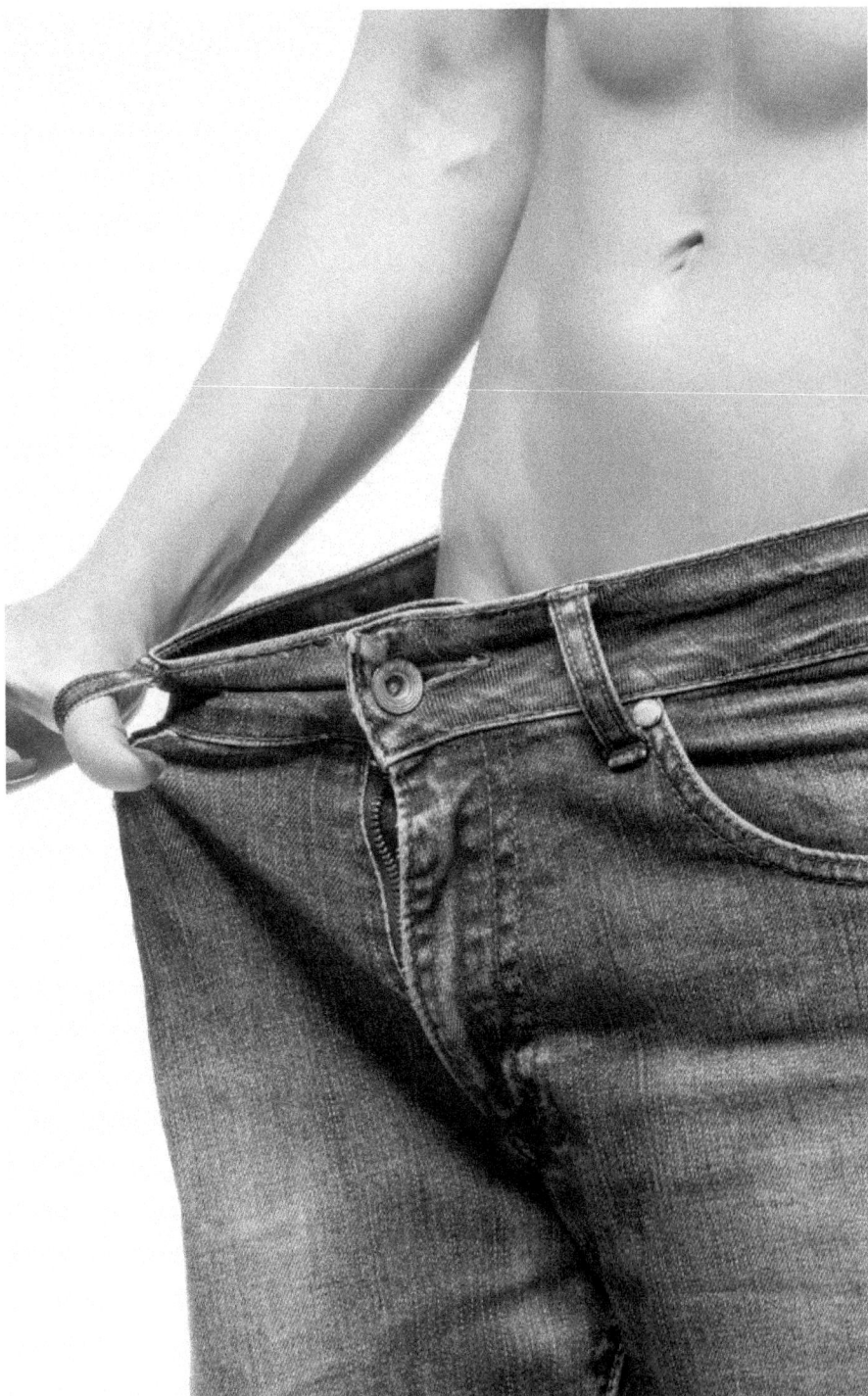

Chapter 4.
How Hypnosis Helps Improve Self-Esteem andConfidence

Y ou've learned most things in your life through the unconscious, for example, how to walk and talk. Likewise, you discovered that you had to behave in a certain way even when you disagreed, or it meant that you lost your rights. Perhaps as a kid, they gave you a sweater that you didn't like as a present, and your parents forced you to put it on and show a good face with which your self-esteem started to drop, or something similar happened that slowly decreased your self-esteem.

Hypnosis working directly with the unconscious mind will help you change your progressive and unsure values.

The relationship of self-esteem with the unconscious mind

The unconscious mind controls quite a bit about how we feel about ourselves.

Our unconscious thoughts may be our best friends, or it may be our greatest critic.

These thoughts are automatic and have firm roots in our minds.

It may be that you look in the mirror and your mind tells you that you don't like yourself.

And is that low self-esteem may be the result of programming that does not help us.

Our automatic thoughts are usually recorded in our brain in childhood due to our experiences and how we interpreted them.

Now, what if you can eliminate or change these thoughts?

Or even something much better, what if our minds could interpret them more positively?

That is the basis of hypnosis to increase self-esteem and confidence.

Using clinical hypnosis, we can access these subconscious and automatic thoughts.

With the power of suggestions, we can begin to break them down and reconsider them. In short, hypnosis can be a powerful tool to attack the root cause of low self-esteem.

Trauma can also have a significant impact on our self-esteem and self-confidence.

Traumatic experiences can decrease our feelings of self-esteem and our sense of confidence. Finally, self-esteempresents on a scale. Others may encounter difficulties in certain situations.

But people with low self-esteem often feel that their sense of inferiority is at a constant level. Theymayexperience and feel:

- Hopelessness or depression

- Boredom or lack of motivation

- I was overly sensitive to criticism.

- Lack of assertiveness

- Listen to a cynical and excessively critical internal dialogue

- Feeling like your life is a failure

Low self-esteem and self-confidence: Can hypnosis help you?

The terms self-esteem and self-confidence often use to talk about the same thing, but they are two very different ideas:

Trust can consider as the internal judgment we make about our abilities or qualities.

I'm good at speaking in public but not singing, for example.

Therefore, I am a confident public speaker.

Self-confidence can change depending on the situation.

That self-confident person before a public speech could be a nervous mess singing at karaoke.

On the other hand, self-esteem tends to stay the same.

And it is a measure of our feelings of self-esteem and self-love.

If you have low self-esteem either in public speaking or singing at karaoke, you have negative emotions.

What causes you to have low self-esteem or poor confidence in certain things?

Self-esteem and confidence make up of past experiences.

We receive many negative and positive messages throughout life, which can impact how we feel about ourselves.

These messages can come from our family, friends, teachers, or even from the media.

And unfortunately, we are more receptive to negative messages because, emotionally, they are more robust.

Neuroscience has discovered that all the experiences we live in are recorded in our brains, creating a neural behavior path.

Depending on the degree of emotional intensity or the experience's repetition, that "neural path" or behavior may influence our behavior more than another.

You Can Improve Your Self-Esteem

- There is hope. You can fix negative thinking patterns in your mind.

- But self-esteem is flexible.

- At different periods of our lives, it can be high or low. We can learn to improve it or make adjustments.

- In other words, we should not condemn our low self-esteem.It is possible to build and increase self-esteem.

Hypnosis to increase self-esteem and confidence

Self-esteem has a decisive influence on everything you do and how you feel. It is the subjective assessment that we have about ourselves as human beings. Our belief in who we are, our abilities, and who we want to be in the future. What we feel about ourselves in the present

Self-esteem is a fully learned personal characteristic, and it is not a birth trait like height or eye color. The experiences and especially the conclusions drawn from those experiences determine the perception that one has of oneself.

"What disturbs people is not things but the impressions they have of them," Epictetus

Issues related to self-esteem usually originate in childhood. Our personal history and relationships with the people around us, parents, siblings, and friends, give rise to our opinion.

We receive all kinds of messages as we grow, affirmative and negative. But for some reason, most humans tend to pay more attention and stick with the negative. Feeling not good enough will continue to affect our adult life.

Another possible source of low self-esteem, especially among young people, is the media's enormous pressure. The images and stories of successful people continue to bomb us. It is a fragmented and illusory vision.

Comparing yourself to these people and feeling unsuccessful and worthless is easy if you don't have the right psychological mechanisms. Good self-esteem is the foundation.

Finally, traumatic events, verbal or physical abuse can affect self-esteem. Being subjected to unpleasant circumstances against our will often cause us to lose confidence in others and ourselves.

We often feel responsible and guilty for things that we have no control over. The image of ourselves, self-esteem, is affected.

Each person is different, and low self-esteem affects people in different ways. If a person feels worthless and worthless, his behavior influences, confirming this vision of himself.

Then you have a series of thoughts and feelings that a person with low self - esteem may experience:

- negative thoughtsaboutyourself

- lack of confidence and security

- feelings of permanent uncertainty and hesitation

- lack of motivation

- the sense of constantfailure

- feelings of inferiority

- feelings of being useless, hopeless, and depressed

- feelings of boredom

- feelings of anxiety and worry permanently about making a mistake

- feelings of vulnerability to any criticism

- thoughts that nothing has a solution and lack of expectations

- lack of assertiveness

- feeling tired and lack of energy

- constant wishes for a better life

The most painful thing is that all these difficulties have repercussions in people who experience low self-esteem. People who struggle with low self-esteem seek the approval of others.

They seek to reaffirm themselves by observing the reactions and comments of those around them to value themselves.

Overcoming low self-esteem means learning to accept yourself according to your criteria without waiting to assess other people.

Hypnosis and Weight Loss - How to Train Your Brain to Burn Fat Fast

The nervous system makes up of your brain, your spinal column, and many interlocking nerves. The nervous system is super powerful and can critically influence your goal of burning body fat as it will determine which fuel is best for your body to use for its health and survival. Let's talk about two zones: red zone and green zone.

Red zone

The red zone is where we live stressed, busy, worried about the future; everything is urgent.

Green area

The green zone is the ideal one to relax so that our body works appropriately for digestion, repair, reproduction.As long as we focus on the green area, it will be much easier for our bodies to lose weight.

How do you know if you are in the red zone? Here are some symptoms:

- You feel stressed most of the time.

- You have cravings for sugar or carbohydrates all the time.

- You don't usually sleep well at night.

- You are tired most of the time.

- You feel that everything is urgent.

- You have digestive problems, and you swell quickly after eating.

- Your hormones are out of balance.

Being in this area will convey to your body that you are not safe, in danger, and need to store body fat instead of burning body fat to survive. So, it is essential to spend less time in this area to have better energy and decrease body fat.

Chapter 5.
Enhance Your Motivation

Your journey is going to start with your motivation level. Many things are possible, but it feels like almost nothing is when you lack motivation.

Getting out of bed morning after morning, trying to find the strength to make it through the day can feel as hard as trying to climb a mountain on some days.

Motivation can be found in many different things, but it will always come from our minds. We're passionate about the things that matter; those motivate us to make it through the day.

The first thing you will want to do to motivate you is to change your attitude into a positive one. When we look at the world through a gray lens, we can easily see everything as terrible. When you hate one thing, that hate starts to grow and spread into other parts of your life.

We can't look at life through rose-colored glasses either, because we don't want to make ourselves ignorant to reality.

We have to look at the world, in our life, head-on, as it is objectively. When we can do this, it will be much easier to take on the new things that present themselves to you every day.

Give yourself time to prepare to be motivated, too, not just time to start the weight loss. First, you have to get in the right mindset. Then, you can prepare for your meal plan and exercise regimen before starting. If you try to force yourself into it, you might sometimes make it even harder to get started.

As humans, we like to be independent. Not everyone is interested in being told what to do, and we sometimes seek to be defiant in ways, even against ourselves. Sometimes in our heads, the things we're being told to do won't be our ideas and can instead simply be the pressures of society, our peers, and our parents.

Their voices can still get so deep in our heads that we will mistake them for our own and easily get frustrated with what we're telling ourselves.

It can seem like an internal battle when you are trying to get motivated. There's the part of you that knows what you have to do, and then there's the voice that's telling you not to do it. To just sit around and wait for tomorrow. Motivation is all about silencing that voice and building one of encouragement.

Don't allow any regret into your life or the future. Shame can be such a wasted emotion. It is not. There is a psychological purpose for guilt. It causes us to look back on our mistakes and question our motives for doing certain things. Regret can teach us how to be better in the future. However, too much sadness can lead to a lot of time wasted.

Some individuals will be so regretful over certain decisions that it consumes their entire life. If you want to move forward and be motivated, not just about weight loss but with everything in your life, you also have to learn how to let go of regret. Feeling it in the first place isn't wrong, but don't entertain it anymore.

Think of it like someone you pass at the grocery store, someone that you want to still is respectful towards even though you aren't very fond of him or her. Instead of talking to them and inviting them out to dinner, simply smile at them and keep walking.

We have to learn to process all feelings of regret and emotions of guilt and shame. Simply let it passes, but do not allow it to stay past its welcome.

You are the person that you are right now because of the life that you've lived. It can be so easy to think, "Oh, I should have done this," or "if only I had gone with the other option." However, if we hadn't made that one choice, then our lives would be incredibly different than what they are now. Each thing we've experienced, the decisions we've made, and the thoughts that we've had these are all like ingredients that go into what makes us who we are. When you can learn to love yourself and the person that you've become, then it will be easier to build that motivation because you'll let that guilt and regret losing.

Look at what motivates you right now, at this very second. What's the first thing that comes to mind? Maybe it is wanting to make a loved one proud or providing for your child. Perhaps your motivation is getting your bills paid or merely making your next meal. Whatever it is, this can tell you a lot about what drives you in this life.

When you can become aware of all the motivating factors in your life, it will be easier to use these images and ideas when you are struggling in certain situations.

If nothing comes to mind at all, then it is time to do some soul searching. At the very least, wanting to make ourselves happy should be a motivator. Feeling good and looking better is all I need to motivate me some days; however, others require a little more work.

Honestly, sometimes food was a motivator for me. I would tell myself that if I could avoid fast food all week and eat healthy Monday-Friday, I could go crazy that Saturday.

I told myself it didn't' matter if I wanted to drive myself through Taco Bell, Wendy's, and KFC all in one week. Whatever I decided for Saturday would be fine, as long as I stayed resilient against my cravings for Monday-Friday.

If I was struggling on Wednesday and just wanted to skip the salad I brought to work and walk to the fast-food joint across the street, I would remind myself that I could get it on Saturday. When I would diet in the past, I would think that I had to cut all lousy food out for the time being. It would drive me crazy! Eventually, I realized that I had to give myself looser restrictions and remind myself that it wouldn't be too long before I could have fast food again. It helped keep me motivated throughout the week, rather than always thinking about the food I wanted.

What would end up happening was that I felt so good about myself for eating healthy all week that I wouldn't want to ruin my streak so I would keep up the diet. I would get to Saturday and think to myself that I had done so well all week, why ruin it now?

I might still occasionally go out to dinner with my family on the weekends and get something that isn't great for me, but then this was a reward. I realized that motivation would breed more motivation. The easier it was for me to get started with the things I want and stay focused on my goals, the more this strengthened my willpower. There will always be hard days, but I remind myself that this is part of the process.

Your Dream Outfit

"Weight loss doesn't begin in the gym with a dumbbell; it starts in your head with a decision." — Toni Sorenson3

Some people will put pictures of their celebrity icons on their fridge, or maybe even their mirror so that they see them when they wake up. You need the motivation to help you picture yourself in your future, not someone else's body and journey.

If your primaryreason is done by comparing yourself to others, that will not be healthy in the long run. Instead, it might drive you to eat more because you are feeling bad about yourself, in more of a fragile state where you will decrease motivation levels.

The thing about celebrity bodies is that if they aren't photoshopped, they were still achieved through trick lighting and a team of makeup artists and a personal trainer and shopper that gives them all the tools needed to lose weight.

Most of us women are doing this on our own, so we have to stay realistic.

If you are 5 feet tall and you put Victoria's Secret model on your fridge, that's not going to do you any good. We all have different bodies, and even if you were at your healthiest body weight, you might still not look anything near to the person you are comparing your body to.

Some of us are naturally curvier as well, while others might be stick-thin. You might have more massive breasts and hips, or a more prominent shoulder structure than many thinner models on the runway.

We can't expect our bodies to look like theirs if the design and height aren't the same, so using other people's pictures is never a good idea.

It can just make you feel worse about yourself because you might get below your healthy weight and still not look like the other person, so you will even be disliking your body.

Right now, think of what your ultimate dream outfit would be. Whether it is a slim-fitting dress, or a cute crop-top and some butt - lifting high waist jeans, think of a company that you want to be able to look totally cute in. It is going to be your biggest motivator when you are getting started. You will be able to see yourself in this dress and be able to look at it with your own body, not just what someone else might look like.

Be realistic with your sizing as well. Only go down a few sizes, somewhere that you would still feel good about yourself getting into. If you are a size 24 right now and buy a size 0 dress, that's unrealistic. That could take years to get into, and there's a good chance that your body structure still wouldn't be able to slip into a 0. It is a small size, and people with a size 0 and have a healthy body weight are usually shorter, so be realistic.

A size 16 dress would probably be an excellent place to start if you are currently 24. And if you are a size 16 now, then a size ten would be right. Make sure you aim for something in between your height and what half of that size would be, give or take a number.

Chapter 6.
Your Future Self

Make sure your hands and arms are resting gently at your sides, with your palms facing upward. Inhale deeply and exhale all the tension from your body and mind. Bring awareness to each body part from your head and face and down to your feet and toes. Whatever stress and anxiety you hold within each muscle, breathe it all out.

Inhale and imagine pure light and energy rushing through you through your nostrils and into your inner self. When you let go of your breath, imagine that all negativity and stress is escaping you, as if you are blowing it out of your mouth. Say this now:

"I am okay. I am thankful for all that my life has to offer me. I can beat my goals today, tomorrow, and every other day in my future. I can overcome fear and frustration. I will not let myself fall. I cannot break."

Inhale deeply and bring your attention to your toes. Feel the air against your skin, your clothes against your body, your weight held safely by the surface below you. Concentrate on what you can smell as you breathe in. Let all the senses take over you and go deep into you internally. Feel all the emotions you felt yesterday, today, and then imagine tomorrow and every coming day filled with joy and happiness.

Let your body relax completely. Listen to the sound around you. The birds were singing outside or the wind howling against your window. Listen to the traffic in the distance or kids playing in the park. Listen to the way your home creaks to the very sound of silence. Let your mind wander, and bring it back to your breath. Breathe in and then release your breath. Say this now:

"I am beautiful not for my looks, but for what I have to offer the rest of the world. I am unique because I try hard. I love every trait about myself because I am worthy of myself. I am independent because I help myself and conquer my fears. I am resilient because I have struggled. It is who I am. It is who I have always been."

Inhale for five seconds. As you breathe in, say to yourself, "This is who I am. It is who I have always been. As you breathe out, notice yourself becoming lighter in your mind and more massive in your body. The surface below holds you gently, embracing all that you are.

You are now one with the universe. You are one in this space. Nothing can hurt you. Nothing bothers you. You are feeling uplifted and motivated to lose weight and gain knowledge doing it. You believe that you can do this with every part of your soul. Breathe in now; this is who I am; this is who I have always been. Breathe out. When I count down and reach zero, you will envision yourself step outside of you, and you are going to stand in front of your ideal weight - your future self. Breathe in. Hold.

Release your breath and all tension you hold in your mind and body. Ten, nine, eight, seven, six, "This is who I am, this is who you are, and this is who I have always been." Five, four, three, two, "This is who I am. I am who you are. This is who I have always been, who you will still be. "one zero.

You are standing in front of your future self now. Who is this person? She is you. What does she look like? She has the same clothing fashion as you do. Her eye color is the same, but her face looks different. It's thinner, and her shoulders and arms are smaller than yours. Her stomach doesn't have what you have, but she still looks the same.

It's as if you are looking at your reflection, except a smaller, thinner version of it. You are both beautiful. It is who you are. It is who you will always be and who you have ever been. There is no difference in action, feelings, thinking patterns. You are looking at yourself and feeling euphoric and happy.

She takes a step toward you now and says, "I know who you are. I am you, and we are strong together. You don't need to look like me to be unique and brave, because you already are. If you try hard, stay motivated, and conquer your fears, you will be precisely this image as I stand before you. Before you reach this point in your success, you must first believe in yourself. You must feel that you can do it within every part of your body, mind, and soul.

You must reach internally and stay patient and secure for all that you are because we are the same. There is no you without me, and there is no me without you. You will get here. I believe in you. Now believe in yourself."

You breathe deeply now, feeling your body and mind as light as a feather. With every part of your being, you hear what your future self says to you, and you believe it.

When you breathe out, you feel the weight of the world that's been holding you back drain away. You want this most. You believe you can achieve this goal. She reaches out and softly strokes your cheek; her thin fingers and soft palms feel exactly like your own.

You think to yourself, "This is me. It is who I have always been. She is who I will always be. I am beautiful and strong. I am confident and real. If I want to look like this, it will take work, passion, strength, resilience, and motivation to get there. I already am all these things without trying, so I can, I will become her." Your future self takes a step back and says, "I believe in you, now believe in yourself.

I know you want that, and you know you can get there. Be kind to yourself and make time to be just you. I am going to walk toward you now and count to zero.

When I get to zero, I will be inside you and help you overcome all the struggles you have been facing. I will bring positivity and joy into your mind so that you can reach all your goals. We will be strong together for each other."

Ten, she takes a step forward, nine, and another, eight, another, seven, she is five inches away now, six, one-inch closer. Five, four, three, two, one, she has stepped into you now... zero. You have become one together. You feel a burst of energy enters your body. You were strong before, but you feel more robust now.

You were motivated before, but now you feel like you could do anything, and you will. You and your future self-belief in what you can do, who you can become, and where you will go. You two will conquer all barriers that stand in your way.

Take a breath now for five seconds. Bring your attention from within you to yourself now. You feel entirely uplifted and optimistic. In this present moment, you are back to yourself and the weight you are at. You know and have always known that you will look and feel like you just met the future self. You have all the tools to help you, and now even more because you have always been this person.

Say now, "This is who I am. It is who I have always been." Bring your focus now to what you hear. Listen to the sound of silence, the faint humming in the distance, or the creaks your home makes. Return to your physical body, and then wiggle your toes and your fingers slightly. You are one with who you will be, and you are confident and beautiful the way you have always been. Believe that and conquer your goals, because you can do this.

You may open your eyes and continue your day.

Weight Loss Techniques for a Healthy Life

You have to follow fitness routines in your daily life for a balanced life. If weight loss is your aim, you must adopt different strategies to reduce weight. It is not so straightforward in practice when you follow appropriate techniques. You need strict dietary management and preparation to burn your daily calories to do this consistently.

For those who need better results, fitness getaway programs require. There are many ways to lose weight, so you should pick the right one for your health and fitness. Any wrong choices in this regard will lead you to difficulties.

My question is: can you raise the weight on your own? Some of you would say I would quickly, but it is virtually impossible because of our busy schedules. Perhaps we'll pursue this for a few weeks, then we forget about it. The only way you can adopt such successful weight reduction strategies is by fitness centers and visiting training camps to lose weight. You find the whole wellness relaxation package that best suits you during your wellness holidays.

It is an inclusive outdoor wellness package that provides all workout services such as fitness centers, workout retreats, and a regular gourmet meal. The fitness centers have a team of professionals who advise you on various weight loss practices and ensure that your body reacts appropriately.

Remember that the technique you adopt for weight loss will make you safer and not build any other conditions. And to prevent these issues, you should choose a delicious and nutritionally balanced meal plan, which will keep you happy in every way. And once you're done, the next question will be the different forms of weight loss programs. Such tips for weight loss vary from person to person, and the one better for others may not be right for you. Your preparation methods focus on your fitness. When you are an elderly citizen, you domost sports like swimming, biking, and cycling. The spa treatment is another best method to quickly reduce your weight, allowing your mind and body to smooth and comfortable.

Various physical exercises in the weight loss camps practice, and the combination of all these strategies will soon raise the weight. The weight loss camps offer luxurious wellness resorts and programs according to your desire and ensure that you are happy even in your accommodation. You certainly have to follow some useful weight loss tips to make you comfortable in any respect if you are worried about your extra fat accrued on your butt.

Chapter 7.
Mistakes to Avoid

Mistake # 1: Deleting fun foods

"I never take cheese,""I stopped chocolate completely,""Unthinkable to have sweets at home." These little declarations of war, we have heard them all, even pronounced. However, determination is not the key to lasting weight loss.

Mind control over food is the fundamental error, arguably the heaviest and also the most common.

By deciding not to eat the square of chocolate that you adore, you switch to cognitive restriction.

Nutritionist, In other words, it's the start of a relentless match against your body.

And this control is fragile. A smell, tiredness, a blow of depression is enough to overcome it, sooner or later. Above all, instead of learning to recognize hunger, satiety, gustatory pleasure, you are moving away from natural sensations.

We can even end up filling our need with a dish of green beans to succumb to prohibited food.

At the time of "cracking" (hearty dinner, snack, etc.), we enter a vicious circle:

1 / "I shouldn't, I'm going to get fat."

2 / "I will not eat more of the week."

3 / "I overeat before being deprived of it."

Not sure, moreover, that this pattern is not repeated for several days in a row. What is more, the experience of two American researchers shows that we will eventually gain weight. According to their results, after a snack (a milkshake), the people tested spontaneously adjust, without calculation, their next meal portions. What the "restricted eaters" are incapable of.

The solution:

No longer believe in "foods that make you fat." For this, the nutritionist recommends an exciting exercise. A person who always ends lunches and dinners with yogurt or fruit, perceived as "authorized" foods, can replace them with two squares of chocolate, the famous "prohibited" food. By keeping this rhythm for six days (weighing before and after), she will have lost weight or, in any case, will not have gained it! In terms of calories, the two squares of chocolate (dark or milk) are below the intake of fruit or yogurt. Result: chocolate will no longer be a "devilish" food.

The person will even find the desire to eat fruits and dairy products because they are right and not because they "make you lose weight.

Mistake # 2: Obey the rule of three meals a day

We have been told enough to believe it: you have to eat three meals a day. Better still, a king's breakfast, a prince's lunch, and a poor man's dinner.

The golden rule is much simpler and natural: you have to eat when you are hungry.

We just haven't shown a relationship between the number of meals a day and weight gain.

Then, a morning calorie is the same as that of midday or evening. Studies have not shown that the body would assimilate cheese, butter, fish, fries, yogurt, fruit, protein, etc. differently depending on the time of day, which has been observed in people who practice Ramadan.

"They consume the whole day's food ration all at once, even in the evening or at night. However, after a month on this diet, they do not gain weight unless they are too rich.

The solution:

It is up to everyone to see whether they need to eat in the morning or not, a lot or a little. However, not forcing yourself to breakfast does not mean allowing yourself to throw yourself into anything at 11 am in the cafeteria or bakery. If the stomach is starving, it is better to wait until lunch while crunching an apple or taking a banana.

What your brain will deduct itself from the next meal. Be careful, however, to make the difference with snacking! We eat because we are hungry. We snack because we want to eat. But small snacks are often minimized.

Mistake # 3: "Believe" in light

Consumption of these products has only increased. Have people become less fat? No. "We now know that light and sweeteners will not solve overweight, obesity, and diabetes.

Diet products only "flatter the brain": you know you are eating a lower calorie product. But you lose in pleasure what you gain in satisfaction. A dietary cookie, "to taste, it's no longer a treat. And the 10 to 15% fewer calories compared to a normal cookie will not make a major difference, "he continues. Not to mention that, when it comes to salty snacks, "the lightened diet had the effect of distorting our taste," notes the nutritionist. Bread crumbs with fish flesh and a little oil nothing to give us spontaneously want".

The solution:

The war against sugar is no longer necessary. To his patients, Dr. Cohen advises instead to keep it, choose real sweets, and, for drinks, coffee or tea, add Stevia, a natural sweetener, for the most addicted palates with a sweet taste.

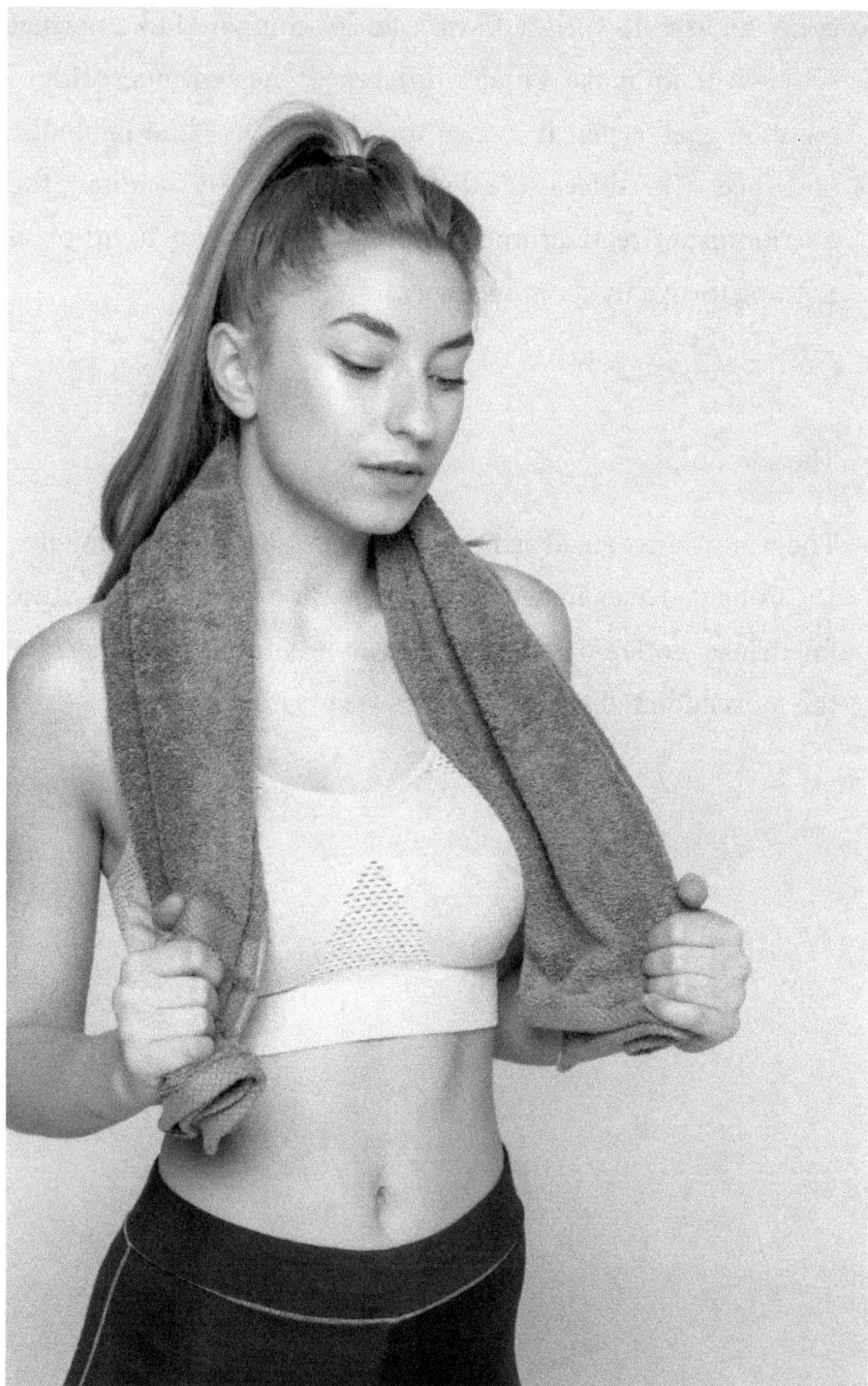

Chapter 8.
What is A Gastric Band?

The Gastric Band is a hypnosis process used to change the lives of seriously overweight and obese people who've been unsuccessful at reducing weight using other techniques. It replaces the actual Gastric Bypass Surgery with a hypnosis-based different focused on achieving the very same result of reducing the quantity of food the stomach can take in one meal. While this sort of surgery of the mind is not new, its weight loss application is unique.

Researchers worldwide agree that one of the keys to wellness, health, and individual growth depends on understanding the mind/body connection.

Gastric band hypnosis is more secure and less pricey than having the equivalent surgery executed.

How Gastric Band Hypnosis Works

Gastric band hypnosis uses the creative imagination instead of the scalpel to help overweight people restore control over their eating habits. You most likely already know what the stomach band surgeries or fat burning surgical treatments encompass. The procedure executes in a medical facility operating space where a team of cosmetic surgeons and nurses make tiny incisions in your upper body and stomach and slide little surgical tools and electronic cameras right into your inner body.

They cut and shed a tunnel around your stomach and connect a banding gadget that can take off your stomach's top component.

The dimension of this top part of your gut can readjust to make sure that it takes to get just a little amount of food. So, you end up being incapable of eating more than 4 or 5 mouthfuls conveniently.

As soon as this surgery does, if you were to eat more than your new smaller b can hold, you will become physically incapacitated. It is a usual outcome that calls "dumping." It is so common that a wordcreates to describe the feeling.

The surgical treatment is to make it compulsory for you to consume smaller sized amounts of food. Smaller meals will imply more effective weight management. However, there isn't assurance that you will finish smaller sized dishes, even if you have had the procedure.

This new weight loss program, gastric band hypnosis, takes advantage of the surgical treatment imagery. Using your creativity, youpersuade that you have had the band dental implanted, and you will respond as if you have had the procedure.

I am leaving you with the capacity to build the brand-new routines that will certainly sustain your new, much healthier way of life for the remainder of your life.

Lately, Gastric Band hypnosis continues to produce waves in the multimillion-pound weight reduction organization, marketing itself as the ground-breaking technique to help people lose weight andmaintain their undesirable pounds away. Individuals have stirred up, be they, common homemakers, to widely known stars using hypnosis for weight decrease to preserve their bodies and help their fat loss.

Like many new weight reduction strategies, individuals ask a fat reduction with Gastric Band hypnosis. This over-hyped dream does not work-like marketed, or can it be the wonder that individuals have been looking for?

The term hypnotherapy often evokes photos of women and men performing absurd methods under hypnotherapists' training to many people. As a result of this portrayal of hypnosis, individuals occur to be slow to try and also skilled Gastric Band hypnosis as a weight reduction technique for his/her weight loss goals. An effective Hypnoband prepare for weight decrease differs from your standard method used by lots of Hypnotists;its tailors at people with a BMI of over 25, not just a couple of extra pounds to lose.

Drop Weight With Hypnotherapy Using Gastric Band Hypnosis

Have you become aware of gastric band surgical treatment? People try it as an excellent way to shed weight, and it does work to ensure, but did you understand that it is a costly strategy.

One susceptible to obtaining a slipped band, indigestion, irregularity, looseness of the bowels, nausea, and throwing up and many others?

What happens if you found a way to have every one of the benefits without the surgery's danger and expenditure?

There is a technique in hypnosis that offers this. Gastric band hypnosis is a new technique in hypnosis where you get ideas that you have had the treatment, and incredibly you will start to act and live as if it were real. It is one of the several ways in which you can slim down with hypnosis.

Chapter 9.
The Concept Of Hypnosis

Understanding Hypnosis

For over 200 years, individuals have been contemplating and contending about hypnosis, yet science still needs to explain how it happens entirely.

We see what an individual is doing under a trance, yet why the individual is doing it isn't apparent. Ultimately, this riddle is a little piece in a lot more giantpuzzle: how the human personality works.

It is far-fetched that specialists within a reasonable timeframe will think of authoritative clarification of the brain, so It is safe to say that the phenomenon of hypnosis will further remain a mystery.

Be that as it may, specialists know the general aspects of hypnosis. As such, they have some examples of how it functions. It is a condition of stupor portrayed by serious suggestive, unwinding, and expanded dream. It is unlike sleep since the individual is alert at all times. On the other hand, wandering off into fantasy land, or the feeling of "losing yourself" in a guide or film, is generally expected.

You are entirely mindful. However, most of you're the environment around you is blocked out. To the close to avoidance of some other idea, you focus seriously on the current point.

Specific occasions can trigger genuine dread, misery, or satisfaction, and in case you're stunned by something (for instance, a beast hopping out of the shadows), you may even shake in your seat. That is why most analysts characterize every single daze as self-trance of sorts.

Milton Erickson, the twentieth century's driving master in sleep induction, contended that people are mesmerized every day. In any case, most specialists focus on the condition of daze brought about by purposeful unwinding and thinking works out. This significant mesmerizing is frequently compared among alertness and rest to the relaxed mental state.

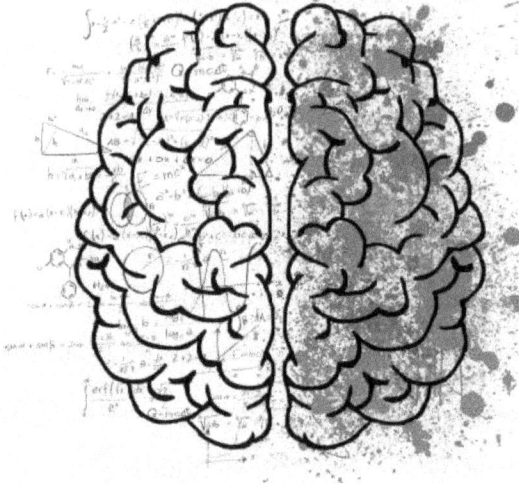

Hypnosis in Psychology

What exactly is hypnosis?

While definitions may contrast, the American Psychological Association characterizes hypnosis as an agreeable collaboration in which the member responds to the hypnotist's recommendations.

Because of necessary acts, the trance has turned out to be notable.

People urge to direct unprecedented or silly conduct, yet also clinically demonstrated to give medicinal and restorative favorable circumstances, mosquitoes. Hypnosis has even recommendeddiminishing dementia manifestations.

What do you think when you hear the term trance specialist? In case you're similar to numerous people, the term may invoke photos of a vile stage miscreant who, by swinging a pocket watch to and from, makes a sleep-inducing state.

There is little similitude among mesmerizing and these cliché portrayals. "The trance specialist doesn't mesmerize the person, as indicated by analyst John Kihlstrom.

Or maybe, the trance specialist fills in as a sort of mentor or coach whose assignment is to help the individual turned out to be mesmerized."

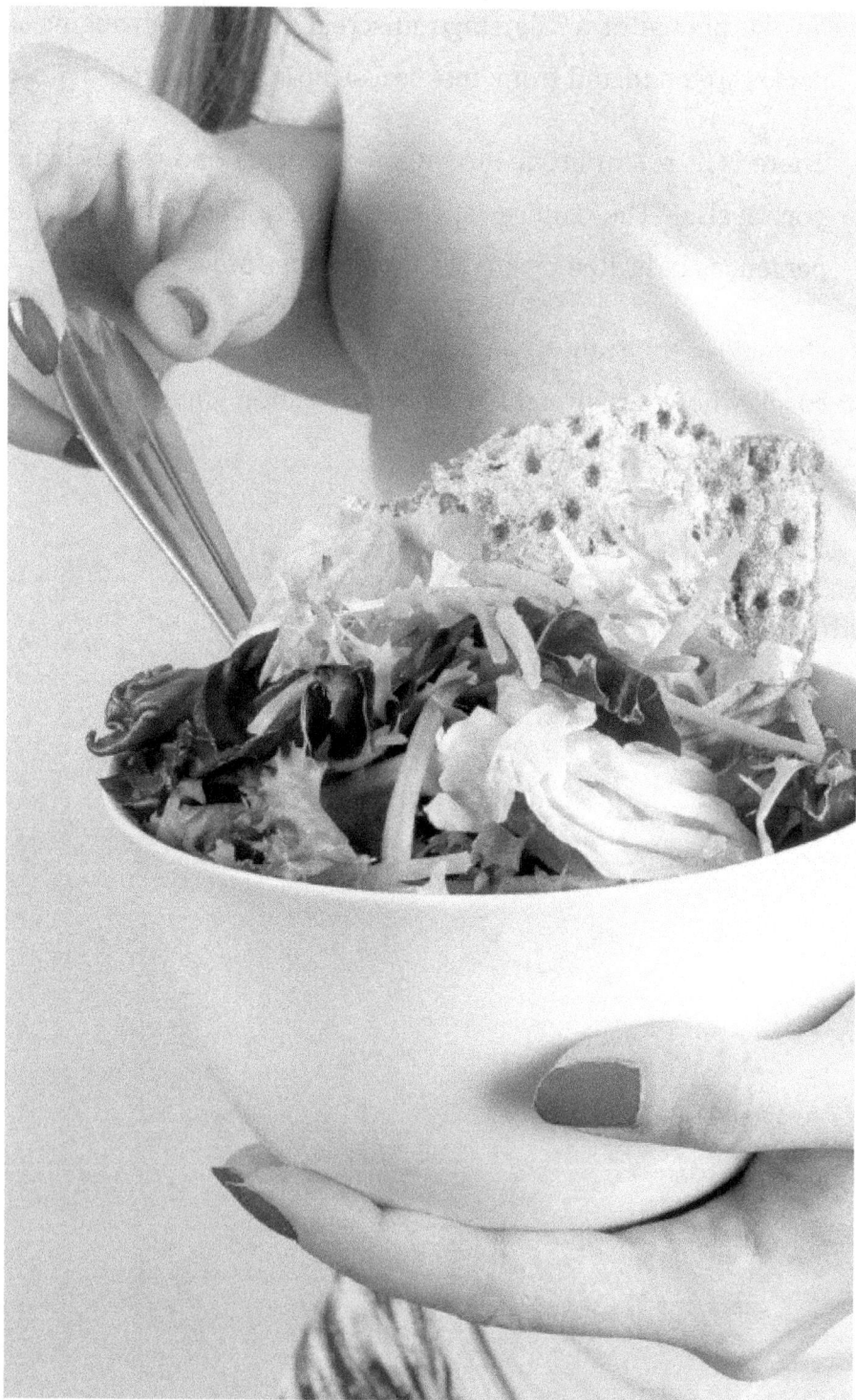

Chapter 10.
An Overview Of Gastric Band
Hypnosis

What Is A Gastric Band?

Astomach band is a silicone flexible apparatus utilized in weight reduction medical procedure. To create a modest pack over the gadget, the band puts around the belly's upper part. It restrains the amount of sustenance that can be put away in the stomach area, making eating enormous amounts hard.

A gastric band will likely constrain the amount of sustenance that an individual can expend physically, making them feel full in the wake of eating next to no to advance weight reduction. It is a final hotel for most people who have this medical procedure after endeavoring for other weight reduction systems. Like any medical procedure, there are perils in fitting a gastric band.

Gastric Band Trance

Gastric band tranceutilizes without the perils that accompany medical procedures to help people get thinner. Numerous trance specialists use a two-dimensional system. The first hope to characterize your enthusiastic eating's underlying driver.

Utilizing trance, the specialist can urge you to recall long-overlooked nourishment related encounters that may now influence you subliminally. Before performing gastric band hypnotherapy, tending to and perceiving any unfortunate reasoning, examples concerning sustenance can help.

How it Functions

How gastric band spellbinding works: Using unwinding a trance specialist technique will get you a trance condition. Your subliminal is progressively open to proposal in this relaxed state. Trance inducers are making proposals to your intuitive at this stage. With hypnotherapy of the gastric band, this suggestion is that you have joined a physical band.

The psyche is stable, so your conduct will change as needs be on the off chance that you are subliminal that acknowledges these proposals. More often than not, alongside the virtual gastric band's' fitting,' requests will be created about trust and conduct to help you focus on this way of life move.

Numerous specialists will likewise encourage strategies for self-mesmerizing so you can improve your activity after the session. It is also regularly prescribed to instruct yourself on nourishment and exercise to help physical wellbeing and prosperity.

Chapter 11.
The Power of Visualization

With the hypnotic gastric band, you can use your imagination to control your subconscious mind and your body. Visualizing weight loss means that you're creating the image of how you want to be in your mind.

Visualization is a beautiful tool that triggers your subconscious mind so that you can shape your body to match your mental image.

If you visualize according to the way you're supposed to imagine, you will lose weight, improve your looks, and become more energetic. You have to realize that your emotions and thoughts affect your body, either for better or worse. Negative thinking, fear, anger, worry, and stress, harm the body, which then produces toxins that will drastically affect you. Now, if you are happy, positive, and confident, you will be able to energize and strengthen your body.

Learning how to use your subconscious mind during visualization is for your advantage. It is a mental diet, which you need to incorporate into your weight loss plan. You will be able to experience tremendous success with the hypnotic gastric band in addition to affirmations, and visualization, if you start to eat healthily.

Visualization is an excellent thing because it helps you to overcome overeating and emotional eating. The significance of visualization is not in your physical body but in the feelings of overcoming your obsessions and challenges with your food, weight, perfect body, plagues, and the restrictions that are keeping you on a diet merry go round.

With this hypnotic gastric band, you will realize that visualization is a simple process, and it dramatically helps during weight loss.

Find some frequent moments where you will be able to sit down for several minutes and visualize your slim body.

Ignore all the doubts, worries, and negative thoughts and just focus on the image. Forget your current looks and imagine such a beautiful, slim, and ideal weight. Imagine how gorgeous you look in your swimming suit and the tight clothing you always want to wear.

Visualize how your peers and your family are complimenting your slim body and slim looks. Watch the entire scene as if it is real and happening right in front of you. Feel free to construct the different versions of these instances or your other physical roles like dancing or swimming. Visualize the compliments that you're hearing from people about your slim body, and watch them those people as they admiringly glare at you.

Ensure that the images you create in your mind are colorful, realistic, and real. See yourself in each of these natural and exciting scenes with your ideal weight.

Avoid using words that might destroy all the efforts that you've put into and allow only the thoughts of your ideal weight and shape to come to your mind. Powerful visualizations will work wonders when you practice hypnosis because it makes the mental image a possible reality.

Powerful Affirmations

You should change your lifestyle if you want to have experience permanent weight loss or control. Powerful affirmations are essential in helping to change your lifestyle slowly.

Thus, you should practice regular affirmations for weight loss to realize your dream of losing weight.

Notably, weight control is a direct function of your lifestyle because you are solely responsible for your behavior.

In other words, your value determines by your mental attitude, rest and sleep, physical exertion, your manner, and frequency of eating.

You can use effective weight loss affirmations to be able to initiate these measures from your mind. Thus, you should change your thinking; otherwise, no form of dieting will ever help.

Weight loss affirmations are significant in your mind, as they allow you to become a comfort in your desired weight.

It would help if you also consideredyour affirmations' words to ensure that you focus on the solution and not the problem. For instance, you shouldn't say "I am not that fat" because that is the problem that you're saying.

Instead, you should focus on the solution and say words such as "I am getting slimmer" or "I am losing weight every day."

You are repeatedly repeating these words, which will help show that you are determined to take the bold step of living and fitter life. So here are the words:

I weight _____ pounds: this affirmation states the desired weight in your mind instantly, and as you repeat the words, you are reminding yourself about your destiny and all measures that you should take.

I will achieve my ideal weight to enhance my physical fitness: you are embracing a lighter weight and improving your physical activity.

I love eating healthy food because they help me to be able to attain my ideal weight: This statement promotes healthy eating and cravings for healthy food.

I ease digestion by chewing all my food to reach my ideal weight: This affirmation is perfect to say before every meal because it guides the rate and amount of food you consume.

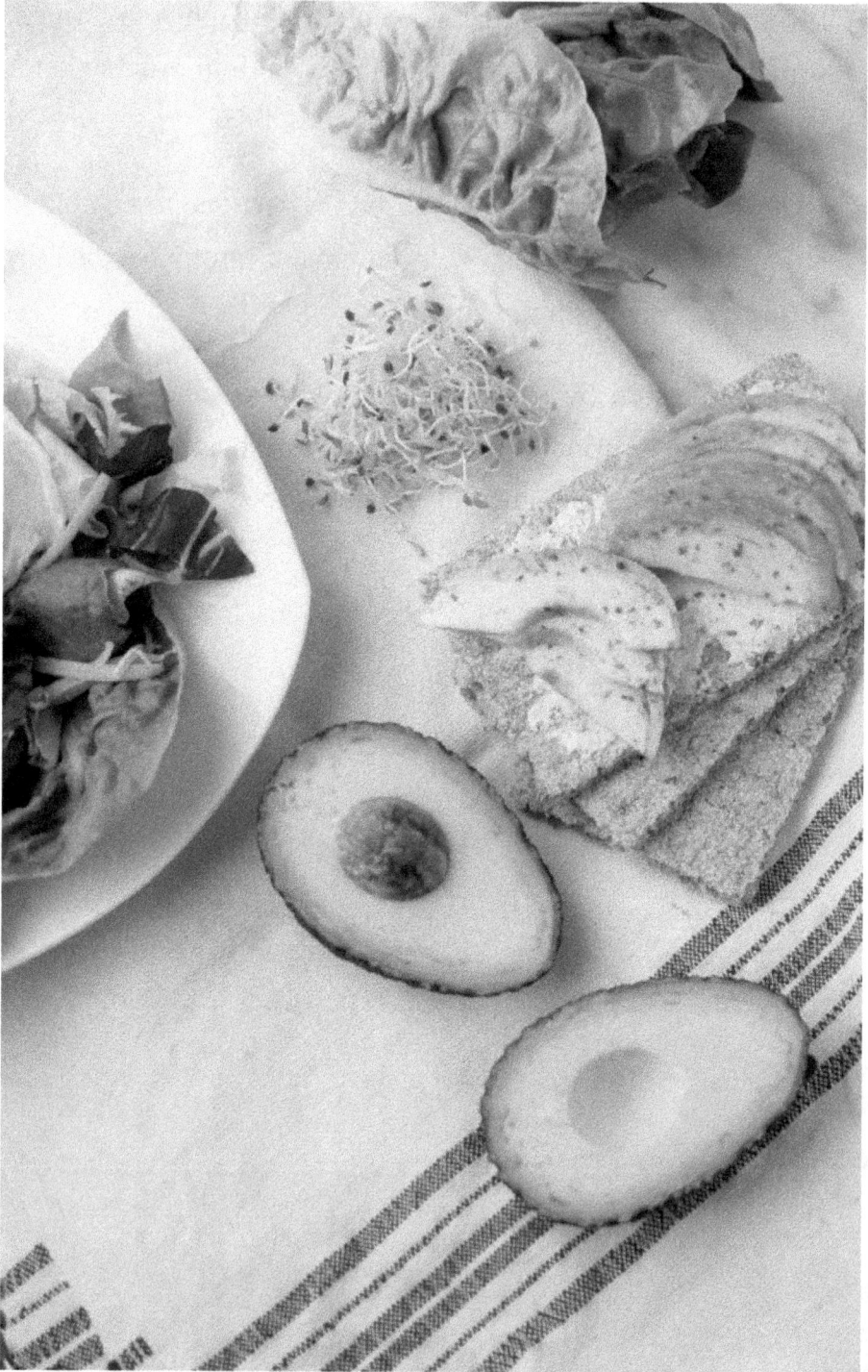

Chapter 12.
Re-programming
Your Mind

The Real Secret ToSuccess

Many psychologists assert that nearly all of our programming is implanted in our subconscious minds at a young age and cannot be changed. They are just about the first part. You've got all types of programming on the mindset there by parents, teachers, friends, media, and culture. A good deal of it had been unhelpful. A good deal of it's still there. Luckily, you can reprogram your mind with new goals and adjust your life direction at any given age.

One difficulty is, you did not receive a user's manual to the mind when you're born, plus they do not teach this stuff in college. Another issue is that even though many more thought leaders are now leading the way to use your mind for behavior change and personal accomplishment, a lot of the advice delivers at a mysterious or pseudoscientific bundle.

It leads to doubt and increases the number of critics that say it is all a lot of nonsense. You will need only look at Olympic and professional sports to observe that psychological training is a serious business. Now, advances in neuroscience and brain imaging technologies like functional MRI, PET, and SPECT scans have continued to confirm psychological training's potency.

You Think Less Than You Think

Did you do something illogical or completely reverse of what you stated you wanted? Subsequently, did you say about yourself, "Why did I do this?" Why can you scarf down a whole bag of biscuits in a yawn as soon as your conscious want is to receive a slimmer and fitter body?

Why can you skip a workout as soon as your conscious desire becomes fitter, healthier, and much more muscular? You are free to choose any actions and make any choice consciously.

Most individuals, however, are entirely unaware of the amount of "automaticity" in the office in their everyday lives. Research by Dr. John Bargh of Yale University indicates that around 95 percent of your behavior chooses. Some specialists believe that the subconscious constitutes as much as 99 percent of your brain's purposes and conscious thinking is only the suggestion of a vast iceberg.

An immense quantity of psychological activity is happening beneath the level of conscious awareness. It feels as if you are willfully picking every action since you observe a thought pop into your mind before you do something.

Your Brain Works Faster Than You Can Think

Do most of your emotional activity occur on the subconscious level, but the subconscious processing also occurs quicker than your conscious mind may think?

Research on subliminal perception has indicated that you cannot consciously find a photo that flashes onto a screen for under fifty milliseconds. However, your nonconscious neurons may perceive it.

Electrical impulses in the mind can shoot in milliseconds, letting you respond to stimuli you haven't consciously discovered. It helps the elite athlete that must perform complicated skills with accuracy. Additionally, it helps in everyday circumstances where you have to make split-second decisions or act fast to keep you from harm's way.

Sadly, this might also explain why you do things like overeat or skip workouts. Research by William Gehring and Adrian Willoughby at the University of Michigan discovered that unconscious processing happens so quickly that spontaneous decisions can make without consulting with your conscious mind.

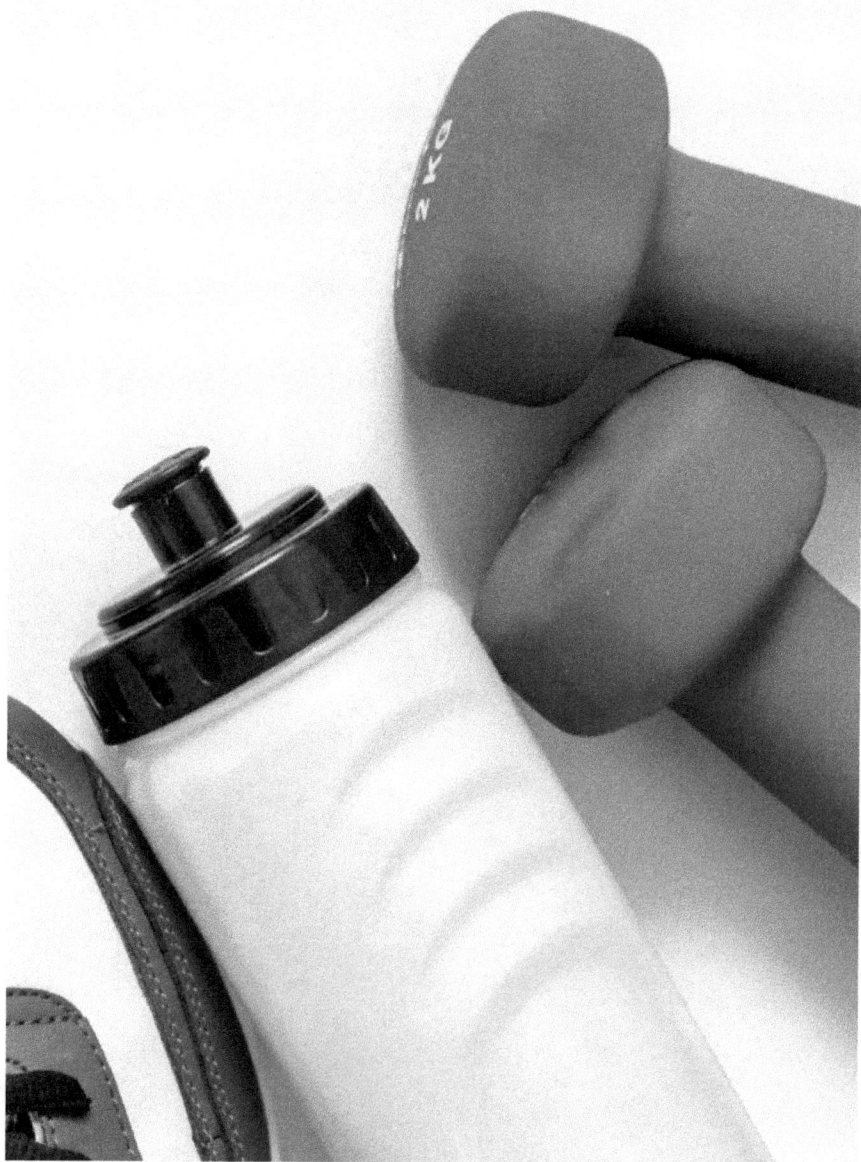

Chapter 13.
How Gastric Band Hypnotherapy Works

The Hypno-Gastric Band Procedure And How It Works

To improve the therapy, the software I use consists of four sessions and two take away tapes. The first three sessions have a length of up to 90 minutes and take place every week. The last session is a follow-up session four weeks after the third session and lasts 50 minutes.

In addition to conducting the Hypno-Gastric Unit's actual 'surgery,' we develop new patterns through this procedure that will help your lifestyle and healthier food decisions and explore long-forgotten memories around food that may influence you subconsciously. The intention is to recognize your emotional eating as the root cause.

During a simulated gastric band treatment, the acts mean to signal your subconscious mind that you have had actual surgery. In a deep state of relaxation that takes you into hypnosis, this is conceivable. Your aware rational mind circumvents, and your subconscious mind is more open to new thoughts that are valuable to you.

You must listen to the recordings you will get from me during the program. They will help you stick to and sustain your lifestyle improvement.

I will help you through every stage of the program and explain what happens at any stage.

In certain situations, as part of a weight reduction regimen, it may be essential to continue hypnotherapy sessions after the treatment. It may be useful for overall wellbeing to resolve any psychological concerns that may be present.

The entire process is a fun, calming experience, and you can feel calm after every session.

Hypnotherapy is a very successful strategy for modifying patterns and attitudes, interacting with challenging feelings and fixing unresolved difficulties. Your performance is entirely up to you and your determination. You are most likely to receive positive outcomes if you believe in the procedure and support the therapist.

The process itself is very straightforward, and all you need to do during our hypnotherapy sessions is to follow my directions, contribute, and listen to your recordings. During our hypnotherapy sessions, getting relaxed and trusting is essential. Investigating a therapist and scheduling a phone meeting to find out more before you agree is sound practice.

Does Gastric Band Hypnotherapy Work?

There are also success stories of people with gastric band hypnosis who have lost weight, such as this one published in the Daily Mirror.

A more complicated picture is given by another article here in the Irish Times.

It provides a few exciting suggestions on incorporating this intense type of hypnotherapy care that I want to repeat and highlight success stories.

Gastric band hypnosis used in a once-off treatment alone will not be adequate to help you resolve the weight dilemma.

Itutilizes a thorough hypnosis program for weight loss that discusses all facets of the weight dilemma in a tailor-made form for you as a person.

What Do I Mean By That? Let Me Explain.

In a hypnotic trance state, simulated gastric bypass surgery will be carried out so that the ideas will sink into the subconscious mind. If they soak in for a little bit, by guiding you to eat smaller servings, your subconscious mind can help you lose weight.

Do not expect your waking mind to be persuaded that you have undergone surgery. You are not going to be that. It's not got to be. In the phase, it is not what matters.

Instead, change your mindset and aspirations to look like a weapon, as a means to an end, at the virtual gastric unit. The effects of the medication on the subconscious mind and the adjustments you make to your post-treatment lifestyle are what matters.

You are ideally prepared to get the most out of your care when you follow this realistic mind style, so you may not get side-tracked by the inbuilt censors of your subconscious.

Chapter 14.
Preparing Your Body For Your Hypnotic Gastric Band

T he physical gastric band requires surgery, which involves reducing the stomach pouch's size to hold less food, and because the stomach wall stretches, it sends a signal to your brain, so you need to stop eating.

The hypnotic gastric band also works in the same manner, although, in this case, the only surgical tools you will need are your mind and your body, and the significant part is, you can conduct the procedure yourself. The hypnotic gastric band also conditions your mind and body to restrict excess food consumption after very modest meals. There are three specific differences between the surgical (physical) and hypnotic gastric bands:

- In using the hypnotic band, all necessary adjustments do by continued use of trance.

- There is an absence of physical surgery, and therefore you are exposed to no risks at all.

- Compared with the surgical gastric band, the hypnotic gastric band is cheaper and easier to do.

How Hypnosis Improves Communication between Stomach and Brain

How would you know when you have had enough to eat? Initially, you will begin to feel the weight and area of the food. When your stomach is full, the food presses against and extends the stomach well, and the nerve endings in the stomach's walls respond.

When these nerves stimulate, they transfer a signal to the brain, and we get the feeling of satiety.

As the stomach fills up and food enters the digestive tract, PYY and GLP-1 are released and trigger a feeling of satiety in the brain that also prompts us to quit eating.

The Power of The Gastric Band

A renowned and dramatic case of hypnotic power to influence our bodies directly is in the emergency treatment of burns. A few doctors have used hypnotic to accelerate and improve extreme injuries and reduce the excruciating pains.

If somebody seriously burnt, there will be damage to the tissue, and the body reacts with inflammation. The patients hypnotize to forestall the soreness. His patients heal quite rapidly and with less scarring.

There are a lot more instances of how the mind can directly and physically influence the body. We realize that chronic stress can cause stomach ulcers, and a psychological shock can turn somebody's hair to grey color overnight. In any case, I especially like this aspect of hypnotism because it is an archived case of how the mind influences the body positively and medically.

It will be somewhat of a miraculous event if the body can get into a hypnotic state that can cause significant physical changes in your body. Hypnotic trance without anyone else has a profound physiological effect. The most immediate effect is that subjects discover it deeply relaxing.

Cybernetic Loop

Your brain and body are in constant correspondence in a cybernetic loop: they continually influence one another. As the mind unwinds in a trance, so too does the body. When the body grows, it feels good, and it sends that message to the brain, which thus feels healthier and unwinds much more.

This procedure decreases stress and makes more energy accessible to the immune system of the body. For example, burns patients realize they burn, so they don't need to deny the glaring evidence of how burnt parts of their bodies are. He practically hypnotizes them and requests that they envision cold, comfortable sensations over the burnt area. That imaginative activity changes their body's response to the burns.

The enzymes that cause inflammation are not released, and accordingly, the burn doesn't advance to a more elevated level of damage, and there is reduced pain during the healing process.

What Makes the Hypnotic Work So Well?

A few people think it's difficult to accept that trance and imagery can have such an extreme and ground-breaking effect. Some doctors were at first distrustful and admitted that his patients more likely than not had fewer burns than was written in their medical records because the cures he effected had all the earmarks of being close to marvelous.

It took quite a long while, and numerous exceptional remedies were generally understood and acknowledged before such work.

Once in a while, the cynic and the patient are the same individuals. We need the results, but we battle to accept that it genuinely will work.

Our minds are very much aware of the contrast between what we imagine and physical reality at the conscious level. In any case, another astounding hypnotic marvel shows that it doesn't make a difference what we accept at the conscious level since trance permits our mind to react to a reality that is independent of what we deliberately think. This phenomenon classifies as "trance logic."

Visualization Is Easier Than You Think

The hypnotic we use to make your gastric band uses "visualization" and "influence loaded imager." Visualization is the creation of pictures in your mind. We would all be able to do it. It is an exciting part of the reasoning. For instance, think about your front door and ask yourself which side the lock is on. To address that question, you see an image in your mind's eye. Influence loaded imagery is the psychological term for genuinely significant pictures. In this process, we use images in the mind's eye that have emotional significance.

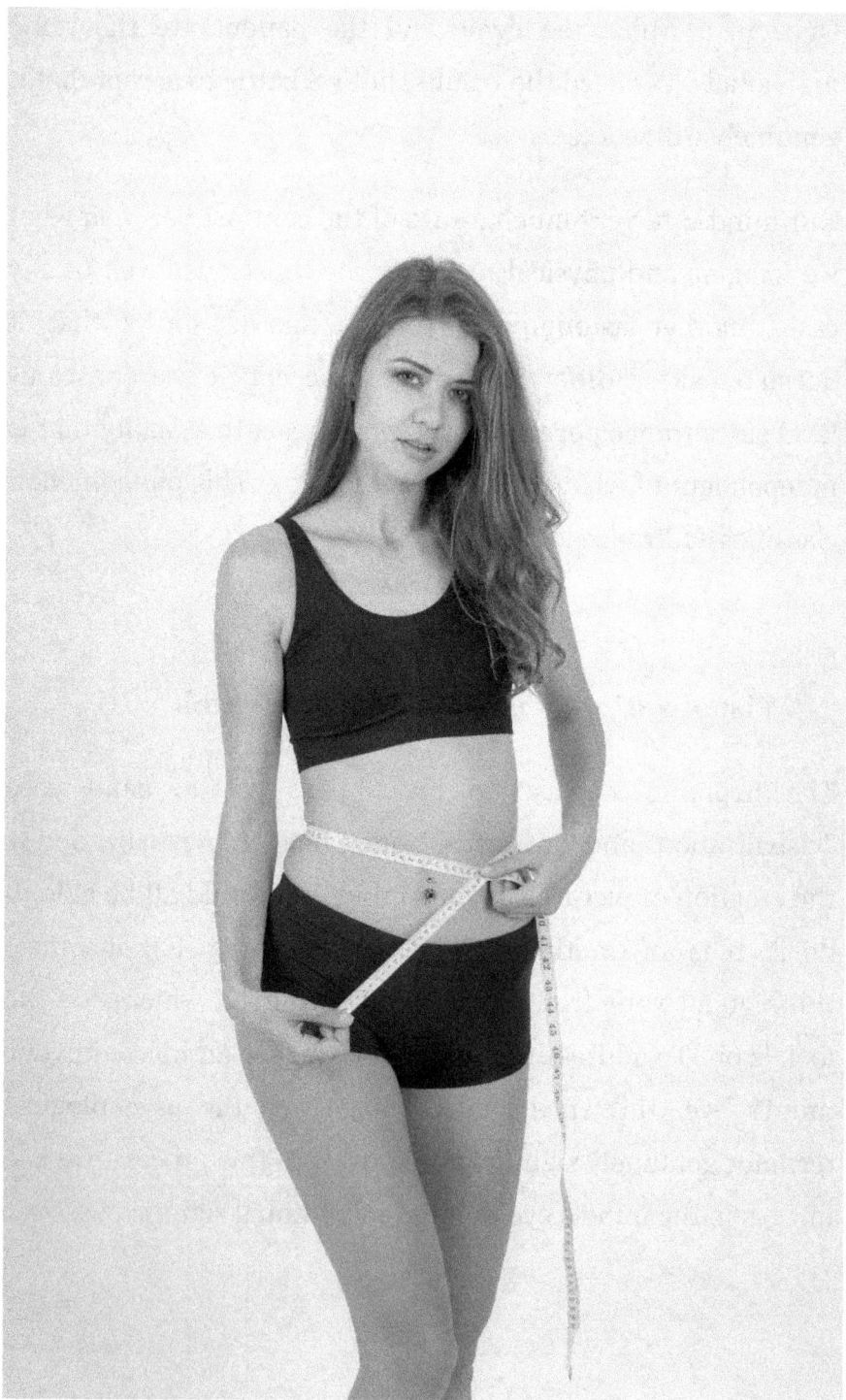

Conclusion

Ultimately, hypnosis, both in a professional or home setting, has the potential to help with weight loss. According to Vanderbilt University, hypnosis works best for individuals who need to lose low-to-moderate amounts of weight.

It doesn't mean that you shouldn't attempt it, but talk with your doctor about working it into a routine that incorporates other weight loss behaviors.

It requires the various number of hypnosis sessions by a hypnotherapist. It may take a long time before professional therapy alters your attitudes and actions, and it may take a while before changed behaviors become a habit.

Any one of these can help you relax while also encouraging you to fall into a weight loss mindset. Make sure you are placing yourself in a place where you can do these meditations safely.

Try not to drive with them, and regardless of whether you're taking a plane or other transportation where another person is in control, be cautious. When you do meditation, always do it at home in a safe place. Possibly, you will fall asleep without realizing it.

After you've attempted a few different reflections, you can use these methods on planes or anywhere else you may go if you know that you can stay awake and alert once you've come out of the meditation or hypnosis.

Recall that the meditations won't make you magically get more fit. They will help you get into the correct mindset necessary to finish the diet or exercise routine you are attempting. They will also assist you with relaxing and decreasing the pressure that can make this procedure harder.

Whatever strategy for eating healthy you may pick, these meditations and trances will help you stop gorging and think it is easier to eat healthily and practice naturally. Recollect that it takes over one attempt and that you should practice it regularly, not once a month. When you can incorporate these snapshots of relaxation into your routine, it will help them work better.

CPSIA information can be obtained
at www.ICGtesting.com
Printed in the USA
BVHW041028040621
608822BV00006B/1549

9 781803 003405